Intermittent Fasting

A Beginner's Guide to Intermittent Fasting

By: Bring On Fitness

© Copyright 2018 – Bring On Fitness – All rights reserved.

information contained within this document, including, but not limited to, errors, omissions, or inaccuracies.

About Bring On Fitness

Our passion for fitness gave life to **Bring On Fitness**. We started with the goal of helping as many people as we can. To educate, motivate and to help change peoples lives for the better. Bring On Fitness is not only for the fitness enthusiasts, but also for the beginner. We strongly believe nothing is more important than learning the basics and creating a strong foundation in both nutrition - through meal planning, and in exercise - by following a specific plan. This is just as important for the beginner, as it is for the experienced athlete.

We set high standards for ourselves, the information we share, and the products we carry. Our goal is to provide you with exceptional products that suit your needs and the knowledge and motivation to help you work towards and achieve your health and fitness goals.

Keep up to date by liking us on Facebook and Instagram @bringonfitness

And for a complete list of reads and a FREE GIFT check us out at: www.bringonfitness.com

"Our Mission is to have a positive impact in changing peoples lives. We will deliver the best possible fitness and nutrition solutions that will empower people to achieve their health and fitness goals."

Table of Contents

Introduction

In the last several years, fasting has been catapulted into the health and fitness limelight – and for good reason! More than just being a purely spiritual practice, as it has been for many centuries, science has shed light on its health and aesthetic benefits. Over the last 10 years or so, many people from all over the world have achieved much better health and fitness by regularly fasting.

In this book, you'll learn about the benefits of intermittent or regular fasting, the different ways you can fast intermittently for better health and fat loss, and other things that can help you make the most of intermittent fasting. When you've finished reading this book, you'll be in a very good position to start fasting intermittently for greater health and fitness. So turn the page, and let's begin exploring this wonderful thing called intermittent fasting.

Chapter 1: The Basics

Fasting is an eating practice that has been around for a very long time. Many people who fast on a regular basis do so in order to connect at a deeper level to their specific deities of worship and in the process, get to know those deities more, as is the case with millions of Christians, Muslims, and Jews, among other religious groups. Some people also fast, believing that it's a way to twist the arm of their deity so that they will get what they are praying for. For atheists or agnostics, fasting is done regularly as a means to further strengthen their self-control and their willpower. Well, actually, even religious people use fasting to develop greater mental and emotional fortitude.

However, recently – and by that, I mean the past several years – fasting has evolved into another form that's neither spiritual nor character-related. It has become a fad diet, i.e., an eating strategy for losing weight and getting into much better shape. For the weight-loss people, they use fasting as a relatively quick way to drop those unwanted pounds. This type of fasting is called intermittent fasting or IF.

Intermittent Fasting

IF is a fasting practice that's quite different from the religious or personal growth kind of fasting because it's not done once a month or once a year only, like Muslims do every Ramadan season. The word "intermittent" implies that it's a regular or frequent type of fasting. How frequent? It can be daily or, at the least, once a week, depending on the type of intermittent fasting performed, i.e., protocol. Unlike the spiritual or personal growth versions of fasting, which are more of a disruption in people's regular eating patterns, intermittent fasting is an integral part of people's lifestyles. In short, intermittent fasting isn't a disruption to one's normal eating pattern because it becomes the normal eating pattern. There are generally four different ways by which intermittent fasting is done – more commonly referred to as protocols – and we'll get into detail concerning these in the succeeding chapters.

How Intermittent Fasting Works

The human body behaves in very different ways when in a state of nutritional lack and when in a state of nutritional abundance. When we eat, our bodies normally need several hours to efficiently and fully digest all the food we consume so that this can be converted into a usable form of energy for optimal function. When we eat just enough food, we have enough energy for normal performance, which means our bodies will have to store extra energy as body fat or burn body fat to compensate for the lack of energy.

Intermittent fasting is a means by which you will deny your body food and, consequently, energy from outside sources so that it will be forced to use your body fat as an alternative source of energy. This can lead to significant weight loss, and if done in conjunction with a good regular exercise program, you can lose even more body fat and weight.

Why You Should Fast Intermittently

Intermittent fasting isn't just an effective way to lose weight; it's a very practical one, too! Why? Most weight-loss diets will require you to be anal about the calories you consume on a daily basis, both on a total and macronutrient level, i.e., carbs, protein and fat. If you've been on diets that require you to watch your calories closely, you know how cumbersome that can be, right? This is not the case with intermittent fasting. With IF, there's no need to count calories or to eat the "right" kind of calories and nutrients from "exotic" foods. Intermittent fasting isn't just practical from a preparation and implementation standpoint but also from a financial standpoint. This means you can make your body slimmer and your wallet fatter! What a great exchange!

For me, an even greater benefit to fasting intermittently is generally better health because truly, health is wealth! Some of the scientifically established health benefits of fasting intermittently include:
   - Improved cellular, gene and hormonal function;
   - Improved cellular repair;
   - Better brain health;
   - Better heart health;

- Reduced levels of oxidative stress, which is a leading cause of cancer;
- Decreased inflammation; and
- A healthier and longer life.

With all the fitness and health benefits of intermittent fasting, don't you agree that it's a nutritional approach worth trying? If you're convinced as I am that it is worth a shot, you'll learn more about the four different intermittent fasting protocols in the next four chapters. Just to level your expectations, none of the protocols are perfect. Actually, nothing in this world is perfect. Each protocol has its own strengths and limitations, which will make one protocol or other much more suitable for you than the others. So if one protocol doesn't seem to work well for you, there's no need to throw in the towel on intermittent fasting. There are three others you can try. Keep in mind that the protocols are your servants and not your masters, so if one protocol doesn't work for you, ditch it for another. You shouldn't fit the protocol; instead, the protocol should fit you.

Chapter 2: The LeanGains Protocol

The LeanGains intermittent fasting protocol was created by Martin Berkhan with the primary intention of reaching an optimal body mass composition, i.e., the ratio of body fat and lean mass to overall mass. One of the things that characterize this protocol is a regular exercise routine (a powerlifting-inspired one) and carbohydrate consumption, which are cycled within LeanGains. This can help you increase muscle mass, reduce body fat levels, and change or maintain your weight while changing your body mass composition.

One of the protocol's strengths is simplicity in terms of being an eating and exercise program. Intermittent fasting is a generally simple way of eating that isn't very particular about the kinds of foods you eat, and the powerlifting-type workouts recommended in this protocol are made up of compound movements that involve more than one muscle group. Compound movement exercises, also referred to as multi-joint exercises, are the simplest and best types of exercises for building muscles and losing body fat.

Implementation

The LeanGains intermittent fasting protocol is a daily type of IF that has two versions: one for men and one for women. If you're a dude, you'll fast every day for 16 hours and eat within an 8-hour window only. If you're a lady, you'll fast daily for 14 hours and eat within a 10-hour window. It's that simple!

When you're fasting, the only things you can consume are calorie-free beverages like plain water, black coffee (either plain or sweetened with a calorie-free sweetener like aspartame, sucralose, or Stevia), natural teas (either plain or sweetened with a calorie-free sweetener like aspartame, sucralose, or Stevia), and diet or sugar-free sodas.

The best way to start implementing this protocol is scheduling your 14- or 16-hour fast starting in the evening. Why? This will make it easier for you to fast because for a big chunk of the time, you're asleep, and by doing so, you can eat for the most part of your waking hours beginning from 6 hours after waking up, which will give you enough energy to do the things you have to do during the day.

Advantages

One of LeanGain's advantages is flexibility. It's easier to fast intermittently with this protocol because you can schedule your fasting and feasting windows whichever way you like. However, I highly recommend sticking to a particular fasting and feasting schedule every day for consistency, which has a couple of benefits. The first is that it becomes easier to turn your dieting into a habit, which won't tax your willpower reserves as much compared to when you change your fasting and feasting schedules from one day to the next. Second, the LeanGains protocol is known to be very helpful in terms of hormone production, which is crucial for getting lean and ripped, i.e., lose fat and build muscle. To be more specific, the protocol is known to be helpful in optimizing the production of growth hormones, which are very important for building more muscle mass and, indirectly, burning more body fat.

Disadvantages

It's flexibility in terms of scheduling your fasting and feasting windows can be offset by the relative inflexibility in terms of food choices. On the days you won't be working out, you'll need to eat mostly protein and fat for increased feelings of satiety, stable blood sugar levels, and increased muscle mass. On the days you'll be working out, you'll need to eat more carbohydrates to fuel your workout and replenish your depleted glycogen stores.

Another possible disadvantage to this protocol is that you'll need to schedule your workouts during your fasting window, which can be quite difficult to pull off when hungry because of the nature of the recommended workouts: lifting weights using mostly compound exercises. You can only break your fast after your workout sessions, which can be taxing on your willpower if done regularly.

Bring On Fitness

Chapter 3: Eat-Stop-Eat

This protocol may be the ideal one for you if you're already eating a healthy diet. If the primary goal of the LeanGains protocol is optimal body mass composition, the primary focus of Eat-Stop-Eat is moderation, which means you're pretty much allowed to eat anything you want in moderate amounts. Have a slice of pizza and not the whole box. Drink a can of soda, not a 2-liter bottle.

Implementation

This protocol is possibly the easiest one to implement because, at most, you'll only have to fast twice weekly without any restrictions on the types of food you can eat. The only restriction is the amount, which is "moderate." However, here's the catch to fasting only once or twice weekly: your fasting periods will be for 24 hours straight. This is possibly the reason for many people choosing the three other protocols over this one despite having to fast only once or twice a week.

If you find the 24-hour fasts a bit extreme, you're in good company. However, the protocol doesn't require that you jump the intermittent fasting gun by fasting for 24 hours immediately. The best way to implement this protocol, especially if you haven't fasted before, is to ease yourself into it. Start by fasting for the first 6 hours after waking up for the first 2 to 4 fasting periods. If you get an average of 8 hours' sleep every night, and you start by eating only after 6 hours from the time you wake up, you will have fasted for 14 hours already! That means you only have 10 more hours of conscious fasting to go! Then, increase the duration by 1 to 2 hours every 1 or 2 succeeding fasting periods until you're able to fast for 24 hours straight.

Again, nothing is off the table when it comes to food on this protocol if only you'll consume them in moderation. It's a buffet in terms of variety but not in terms of amount.

The best days to schedule your once- or twice-weekly fasts are those when you foresee yourself being the least busy, i.e., the least number of responsibilities, obligations, and work to fulfill. The reason for doing this is to minimize your withdrawals from your willpower reserves, which can minimize your risks of quitting or compromising.

While exercise is not a part of this protocol, unlike LeanGains, it's highly recommended that you engage in regular exercise while on this protocol, too, particularly weightlifting exercises. For one, you only need to fast once or twice a week, which means you don't have to work out hungry like in the LeanGains protocol. More importantly, weightlifting exercises can help you burn more body fat compared with aerobic workouts, which means you can exercise for less time and get the same – or even more – fat-burning bucks for your workouts.

Advantages

One advantage of this protocol is flexibility. If fasting for just once or twice a week at most isn't flexible enough for you, never mind if it's for 24 hours per fast, I don't know what is. Also, as I mentioned earlier in the implementation section, you don't have to go on a fast for 24 hours straight when you start. Now that's flexibility!

A second benefit, which should be pretty obvious at this point, is no restrictions as to the kinds of food you can eat – only that consumption should be in moderate amounts. By moderate, I mean an amount that will make you feel neither still hungry nor too full as if your stomach's about to burst. Given that you can eat practically anything at any time other than on your fasting days, your risks of binge-eating and breaking the protocol are very, very low.

Another advantage to this protocol is sustainability. The limited weekly "suffering" significantly reduces your stress and minimizes depletion of your willpower reserves, which means you're less likely to quit on this than the other protocols.

Disadvantages

There's only one major disadvantage to the Eat-Stop-Eat protocol, and that's the long fasting period of 24 straight hours. While it appears to be relatively doable given it's only for once or twice a week, believe me when I say that the relative lack of frequency doesn't make it easy.

Fortunately, there's a way to get this down to pat. As mentioned earlier, the trick is to ease into it and not jump the gun by attempting to fast for 24 hours right off the bat, especially if fasting's something you've never done before. Remember, it's not about achieving your goal as quickly as possible but about achieving it – period!

Chapter 4: The Warrior Diet

This protocol tries to emulate the eating habits or patterns of the world's earliest known warriors, which are the complete opposite of today's smaller-more-frequent-meals approach to healthy weight loss and maintenance. How did the great warriors of the past eat? According to the protocol's proponent, Ori Hofmekler, they purportedly ate two large meals at most daily. Given this theory, Hofmekler recommends fasting every day for up to 20 hours, with an eating window of only 4 hours. Intense, huh? So if you're comfortable with guidelines and rules, the Warrior Diet intermittent fasting protocol may just be the one that's best suited for you.

This protocol is considered a faux-intermittent fast by many legalistic intermittent fasters because of the way "fasting" is defined under the Warrior Diet. For Hofmekler, it's okay to eat small amounts of veggies, fruit, and protein during the 20-hour fasting period. Given that many legalistic fasters define fasting as not eating any solid food, they think this protocol's a joke, but it's worth noting that the Warrior Diet is more about making people eat below their eating thresholds than total starvation. So don't be perplexed with being able to eat small amounts of fruits, veggies, and protein during the 20-hour fasting period.

Implementation

This isn't a very complicated protocol to implement. Basically, all you need to do is eat as much as your stomach can handle for as long as you only do it within a 4-hour window every day. For the remaining 20 hours of the day, you can either eat nothing or stick to very small amounts of fresh veggies, fruit, and protein – and no fruit juice! The ones that come in a can or box from the grocery store - don't count!

Now, isn't that as simple as any diet can get?

However, being simple and unrestricted doesn't mean having no guidelines. The Warrior Diet recommends eating specific types of food during the feasting window because of the belief that while sleeping, our bodies need to get specific types of nutrients in line with our sleeping or circadian rhythms. Another presumption that this protocol makes is that humans are naturally predisposed to eating at night instead of during the day. That's why the Warrior Diet recommends scheduling the feasting windows at night.

To be more specific about the nocturnal benefits of the 4-hour feasting window, timing it in the evening maximizes the parasympathetic nervous system's capacity to let the body relax, calm down, rest, and digest foods completely. What's the benefit to this? It maximizes the body's ability to produce growth hormones, which is key to optimal mass building and fat-burning, as well as optimal cellular repair.

Lastly, you'll need to eat food in a specific order during the feeding window. You'll have to chow down your veggies first, then your dietary fat and lastly protein. If you're still hungry after eating, you can eat more fruit to help you feel full as long as it's within the 4-hour window.

Advantages

Despite the 20-hour fasting period, which is practically the same as the Eat-Stop-Eat's fasting period, many people are drawn to the Warrior diet because the fasting period may be considered as a "faux" fasting one, considering eating small amounts of fruit, veggies, and protein are allowed. This makes the fasting period much easier to go through and the protocol much more tolerable than the others. As a result of being mostly an intermittent semi-fasting protocol, many people find they have more energy even as they lean out using the Warrior Diet.

Another benefit to this protocol, which other intermittent fasting protocols also enjoy, is better sensitivity to insulin. This is crucial for building muscle and burning fat. When your body is more sensitive to insulin, it can process carbohydrates much better and, over time, become more efficient in terms of delivering needed nutrients and calories to your muscle cells. Better insulin sensitivity can also help you gain more muscle mass through better utilization of protein and, more importantly, help you lower your risks of Type 2 diabetes.

Another advantage that the Warrior Diet can give you is lower body fat levels because this protocol can help you to naturally eat just the right amount of food. This is probably due to the fact that you don't have to exercise so much willpower to comply with the protocol and that you can eat to your heart's content during the 4-hour feasting window.

Lastly, the Warrior Diet is a fairly simple protocol to implement. If eating just one huge meal for dinner, a smaller one prior to sleeping, and small amounts of raw vegetables, fresh fruit, or protein during your "fasting" period isn't simple enough, I don't know what is. The simpler a task is, the easier it can be to do it right and, in this case, the easier it is to stick to the protocol, do it right, lose body fat, and become healthier.

Disadvantages

Nothing in this world's perfect, and as such, no protocol is either. However, the good news is that the potential disadvantages of the Warrior Diet aren't so serious.

One possible disadvantage – depending on how you view it – is the "hassle" of having to think of what to eat and the sequence in which to eat your food, both during the feasting windows and during the fasting periods.

Another more serious challenge with this protocol is social in nature. If you love meeting up with friends and colleagues during the day, you might find it quite challenging to stick to the protocol during such meet ups, which will probably involve food and drinks that aren't consistent with the protocol. More than just the food and drinks, you may also have to deal with peer pressure to eat and drink with your well-meaning friends. The Warrior Diet may make you think about where your loyalty lies: your friends and family, or your health and fitness? However, if you're an introvert who loves to spend most of your time alone, this may not be such a big challenge, unlike for extroverts.

The last possible disadvantage or challenge is having to eat most if not all of your daily caloric requirements in the evening in just one meal. If you're used to eating like a bird, i.e., in small but frequent amounts, you might gag at the thought of cramming all that food in one big sitting and a relatively smaller meal just before going to bed. If this is the case, then there's a way you can avoid being overwhelmed.

Just like the 24-hour fasting period of the Eat-Stop-Eat protocol, you can ease yourself into eating all or most of your daily caloric requirements from one big dinner and one small post-dinner meal. A practical way of doing this is to gradually reduce your daytime food consumption and simultaneously increase your dinner consumption by roughly the same amount until you've completely transitioned the bulk of your daily caloric consumption in the evening.

Now, it's possible that you may not fully adapt to getting most, if not all, your daily caloric requirements in the evening because you may not be able to physically chow down that much food in one or two sittings within a 4-hour window. In that case, you can choose foods that have very high caloric density, i.e., food items that contain very high amounts of calories per unit of volume. One of the best food items that pack a whole lot of calories for less volume is medium-chain triglyceride (MCT) oil. You can also go for virgin coconut oil (VCO), which packs a lot of caloric wallop! Simply take a spoonful or two of these oils in the evening to augment any perceived caloric shortfall you may incur if you can't eat that much food within the 4-hour feasting window. The coolest thing about these healthy oils is that they don't affect your blood sugar and insulin sensitivity.

Chapter 5: Fat Loss Forever

If you're the type who craves doing a lot of time in the gym, hitting crazy weights and routines, and loves the occasional diet cheat day every week, this intermittent fasting protocol may just be the most suitable for you. If you examine this IF protocol closely, you'll see that it's actually a combination of the three earlier protocols we discussed: the Eat-Stop-Eat, the Warrior Diet, and the LeanGains protocols. This is because it cherry picks the best features of each of the three preceding protocols.

Implementation

One of the coolest things about this protocol is that you start implementing it with a cheat day, and as soon as you're done with the cheat day, you fast for the next 1 1/2 days or the next 36 hours. After you're done with the day-and-a-half fast, you can choose to do any of the 3 other protocols for the 5 remaining days of your week. That's how your intermittent fasting weeks will be under the Fat Loss Forever protocol.

Advantages

The biggest advantage of implementing this intermittent fasting protocol is you immediately get one whole day of cheat meals once you start your intermittent fasting. By starting immediately with a cheat day, you have something delicious to look forward to, and it can help you launch your intermittent fasting crusade on a very good note!

Another advantage to this protocol is the ability to schedule your days – and to some extent, your circumstances – in a highly flexible manner. This is because you can choose the day on which you'll start implementing this protocol's fasting week and the best IF protocol for the remaining five days of the week in accordance with your schedule and commitments. Given such flexibility, your chances of sticking to it are very high, and along with that, your chances of successfully getting lean or ripped – and staying that way – also become high.

Disadvantages

While the cheat day start may be considered as a big advantage, it can also become a disadvantage if you don't watch it. This is because you run the risk of treating this cheat day as a license to eat inhuman amounts of food and stuff yourself with more food than what you really want to eat or can eat. As with the Eat-Stop-Eat protocol, the main guideline for your cheat days is moderation, which is an amount of food, which, after eating, leaves you neither hungry nor too stuffed. Moderate amounts mean you feel full but not so full. The word "cheat" in cheat days means total freedom to eat "what" you want but not "as much" as you want.

Success Pointers

Consider scheduling your 36-hour fasting periods on days when you're very busy, if you want to optimize your chances of successfully losing body fat. When you do this, your mind will have much less time to think about the fact that you mustn't eat anything for 36 hours because it's pre-occupied with the many things you'll need to do for that particular day. By the time your busy day is done, your 36-hour fasting period is close to being over and done with.

Similar to any other intermittent fasting protocol – or even non-fasting weight loss diets – adding regular exercise into the mix will help you burn body fat much faster. If you want to burn as much body fat as possible within a specific time frame, you should choose a weight-training program over a cardio or aerobic training program. This is because weight-training programs, particularly those that include compound or multi-joint movements like squats and deadlifts, recruit the most muscles with every movement. With such compound weight-lifting exercises, you can burn more calories and, consequently, body fat.

A good weight-lifting program also helps build muscle, which is the most metabolically active tissue in the body. The more muscles you have, the faster your resting metabolism becomes, which means you can burn more fat even while at rest. With a good weight-lifting program consisting mostly of compound movements like squats, barbell bench presses, deadlifts, and overhead presses, you can burn more than twice the calories and body fat in 30 minutes compared to doing cardio or aerobic workouts for 1 hour.

Chapter 6: Getting Started

At this point, have you decided which intermittent fasting protocol to try out? If you have, we have to talk about a couple of other things before you get going – things that can help you start on a great note and sustain your new eating lifestyle.

Mindset

Your mindset about intermittent fasting will determine whether or not your experience will be a great and long-lived one or a short-lived and miserable one. If you're getting into this with the belief that it's going to be very hard and that you'll be in a whole lot of hardship and will basically be living a life of culinary deprivation, then intermittent fasting will be a very miserable experience for you – one that will most likely be short-lived. On the other hand, if your mindset about it is that it's an exciting new world of eating possibilities that can help you achieve that body you've always dreamed of and become much healthier, chances are high you'll have a relatively good experience about it, and your chances of sticking around long enough to achieve your dream body become much higher.

Don't be in a Hurry

While it's true that intermittent fasting has helped many people lose body fat and become lean at a faster rate than traditional weight loss diets, it doesn't mean the results are the same for everybody who has tried IF. First off, intermittent fasting isn't a crash diet because you'll likely be consuming the same number of total calories on a daily basis, but the difference lies in scheduling your caloric consumptions within the day/night. There are several other factors that can influence the speed at which you lose fat, build muscle, or both, like sleep, rest, and exercise. However, rest assured that if you stick to it long enough without going out of bounds, you will lose body fat eventually. As with any other endeavors worth getting into, patience is a virtue with intermittent fasting.

Hydration

Drink lots of water because it will make you feel fuller for longer, ensure you stay hydrated (and feel more energetic), and allow you to exert more effort at the gym, which can lead to burning more calories and body fat. On the other hand, being chronically dehydrated will make you feel "hungrier" and weaker, which can amplify your risks for eating during your chosen fasting periods and eating more than what you really want or need during your feasting windows.

Quality Sleep

If you don't get enough quality sleep on a consistent basis, you'll feel weaker and more sluggish throughout the day. If you feel this way, you'll most likely try to compensate through food and drinks that contain a lot of sugar, which will only make things worse. So do yourself a favor, and get enough quality sleep every night.

What factors determine the quality of your sleep? Two things: duration and depth. You can sleep for 10 hours, but if your sleep is very shallow, you'll still feel as if you didn't get enough sleep the following day. If you sleep very deeply but only for 3 or 4 hours every night, chances are high you'd still feel the same the next day.

A very practical way to get deep enough sleep is to drink a sleeping concoction that I learned from bestselling author Tim Ferriss, who also learned it from somebody else. Mix a tablespoon of raw honey, 2 tablespoons of apple cider vinegar (Braggs, preferably), and a cup of hot water. Drink this concoction before going to bed, and enjoy deep sleep like you've never experienced before. The good thing about this is that unlike sleeping pills, this doesn't make you wake up feeling groggy for the most part of the morning after. More likely than not, you'll wake up feeling refreshed and energized when you drink this concoction prior to hitting the sack at night. Just make sure you get in at least 7 hours of total sleeping time every night to really maximize its deep quality sleep benefit.

Conclusion

Thanks for buying this book. I hope that, more than just helping you learn the essentials of intermittent fasting and how to do it, I was able to encourage you to at least give it a shot. After all, knowing is just half the battle for your dream body and excellent health. The other half is action or application of knowledge.

I highly encourage you to choose one protocol, give yourself a week to plan and prepare your schedule to start implementing it, and give yourself enough time to completely transition into the required fasting period of your chosen protocol. You don't have to apply everything perfectly at once. Start small, and build up your fasting capacity. After all, fasting isn't something that can be easily adapted to. For most of us, not eating is the aberration, and eating is the normal. Hence, it can take some time to fully adjust to intermittent fasting or regularly going hungry, but trust me, it'll be worth it.

Finally, I highly recommend checking with your doctor first before implementing any of the protocols you learned here. While the intermittent fasting protocols are generally safe for most people, it's better to be safe than sorry. You may have an undiagnosed condition for which intermittent fasting may not be suitable, and only by checking with your doctor can you be sure that intermittent fasting can be a very effective health and fitness tool for you.

Thank you, and remember to share how well these intermittent fasting tips work for you. You can do that by writing a review in your Amazon account under YourOrders.

Thank you,

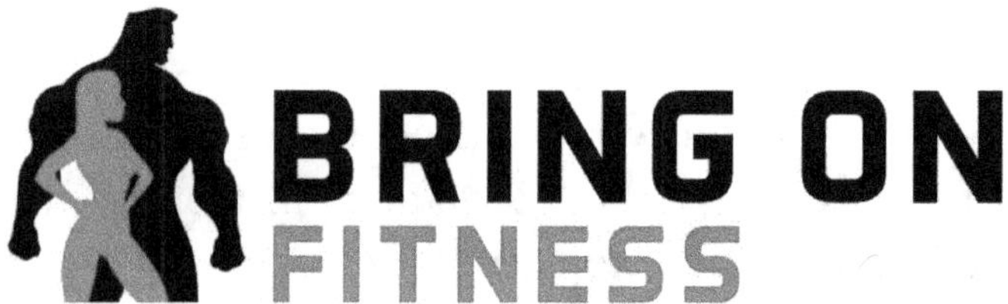

About Bring On Fitness

Our passion for fitness gave life to **Bring On Fitness**. We started with the goal of helping as many people as we can. To educate, motivate and to help change peoples lives for the better. Bring On Fitness is not only for the fitness enthusiasts, but also for the beginner. We strongly believe nothing is more important than learning the basics and creating a strong foundation in both nutrition - through meal planning, and in exercise - by following a specific plan. This is just as important for the beginner, as it is for the experienced athlete.

We set high standards for ourselves, the information we share, and the products we carry. Our goal is to provide you with exceptional products that suit your needs and the knowledge and motivation to help you work towards and achieve your health and fitness goals.

Keep up to date by liking us on Facebook and Instagram @bringonfitness

And for a complete list of reads and a FREE GIFT check us out at: www.bringonfitness.com

"Our Mission is to have a positive impact in changing peoples lives. We will deliver the best possible fitness and nutrition solutions that will empower people to achieve their health and fitness goals."